FREDERICK LOPEZ

SECRETS TO LIVING A HEALTHY LIFE

COPYRIGHT@FredrickLopez2022

<u>LEGAL NOTICE</u>

business guidance. We strongly advise all readers to consult with qualified experts in the areas of law, business, accounting, and finance.

This book is recommended for printing for ease of perusing.

TABLE OF CONTENT

Introduction

Living a healthy life is important for all of us, and paying attention to our own particular health and good has a major influence on the quality of life we can enjoy. Being physically active, eating a healthy diet, taking sensible preventives to insure our particular safety and recognizing the significance of good internal health all play an important part in determining our overall health and good. A healthy life can reduce the threat of developing life- hanging conditions similar as heart complaint and stroke, increase the enjoyment we get from life and help us to live on into an active and healthy old age. A healthy lifestyle is a way of living that lowers the threat of being seriously Ill or dying beforehand. Not all conditions are preventable, But a large proportion or deaths, particularly those from coronary heart complaint and luna cancer can be avoided.

Chapter 1:

Get Healthy-Be A Winner

Synopsis

Just think about what is necessary for you to succeed in your wellness endeavors and in life. You probably will say something like excellent education, brilliant career and a lot of additional things you consider important.

We may agree with everything here, but it's still wise to point out that your health is more important than all of those items put together. If you are physically fit, you can take advantage of all the aforementioned opportunities for instruction, employment, and other things. However, if you are unwell, your only concern will be feeling better, so you won't be concerned about your achievement.

Health Is Key

After determining what is most important to you, you should specify ideal methods for maintaining your ideal weight and fitness level. These are basic guidelines that should be followed daily. Therefore, the task's complexity isn't the main challenge; rather, it's having the self-control to keep moving and not give up before you've even started.

You must first think about your diet. Consider how many sandwiches, chips, and sweets you eat every day and how much damage you are routinely doing to your body. Consider a gradual change to a healthier diet: add more vegetable salads, fish, whole grains, and white meat to your regular meals.

Such foods will be a great source of fiber in addition to being a source of beneficial vitamins and micronutrients. They provide nutrition while also ensuring that your diet contains a range of calories that are safe for your health and weight maintenance.

You might stop worrying about your hips and waist, for instance, as regular consumption of such foods will actually cause you to lose a few extra pounds.

How much exercise you get each day is yet another issue that needs your attention. For instance, you must be even more cautious if you operate in an office. It goes without saying that you must sit at your computer all day long and complete important duties. It's clear that your timetable makes it incredibly difficult for you to fit regular exercise into your schedule. For this reason, we give you a few extra options and suggestions for incorporating more exercise into your daily activities.

Consider simple mistakes like overlooking the lift. Take the steps, and you'll walk more than you might have been able to and get fantastic exercise for your legs. If you only need to travel a few blocks to get to your location, it may be suggested that you drive. Walking outside for ten to fifteen minutes is much healthier for you.

If you consider doing chores around the house as a healthy physical exercise, they won't be a burden. Think of a few more examples. You'll stay healthy, have more energy, and be able to lose weight thanks to this. Your success depends on maintaining fitness in your daily living.

These are merely a few pointers to help you get started on the road to success when it comes to losing weight and getting in shape because being healthy also translates to success in other areas of life. Isn't this what everyone desires?

Consequently, if you are adequately equipped with the knowledge necessary to be successful and fit, you can be sure that you'll find reasonable solutions to any problem. The quality of our existence is rapidly improved in the world we live in by information.

Utilize these instruments to their fullest potential. For your process of becoming effective and fit, they'll be very beneficial.

CHAPER 2

The Facts About Nutrition

Synopsis

Nowadays, you have access to an abundance of nutrition knowledge. Everybody seems to have a different idea of what you should be consuming, from diet books to news articles. There is no denying the crucial role that great nutrition plays in maintaining wellbeing and a healthy weight.

Understand What You Eat

You formerly know how important it's to eat a healthy diet, but you might find it grueling to sift through the information available on nutrition and nutritive options. The" Basic 4" dairy, flesh, grains, and fruits and vegetables might have been a part of your parenting. These nutrient groups have evolved along with the field of nutrition wisdom. What are the introductory nutrient groups? Foods are distributed when they've analogous salutary characteristics. Depending on the diet you choose, you might discover that the food groups are organized else. My Aggregate, for case, has a meat and bean order rather than a meat, flesh, and fish group. To help you maintain your health, then are a many samples of a typical diet.

* Grain cereals, grits, oats, brown rice, popcorn, English muffins, fund chuck , bagels, brown chuck and rolls, whole- wheat pasta, and English muffins.

* Fruit includes apricots, apples, bananas, dates, grapes, oranges, grapefruits, grapefruit juice, mangoes, melon, peaches, pineapples, raisins, strawberries, tangerines, and a fruit drink that's 100 percent fruit.

* Carrots, broccoli, collard flora, green   sap, peas, kale, lima sap, potatoes, spinach, zucchini, tomatoes, and sweet potatoes are some   exemplifications of vegetables.

* Nonfat or Low Fat Dairy skim(fat-free) or low- fat(1), buttermilk, rubbish, and nonfat or low- fat firmed or normal yogurt.

* Flesh and   spare flesh,   similar as beef, pork, game flesh, seafood, and shellfish. Pick only spare meat; remove any egregious fats; repast, poach, or   melee ; and remove skin from flesh.

* Nuts and seeds include almond, filbert, mixed nuts, peanut, walnut, sunflower seeds, and peanut adulation. Other foods include order sap, lentils, and resolve peas. To stay within your calorie needs and encourage excellent health, a healthy eating plan will determine how important of each nutrient group you bear. A sensible diet strategy could also help you in literacy-

* How numerous calories per day you need.

* How important of each mess is considered a serving.

* How to make healthy food opinions for each food order.

Being sluggish? Have you been   passing digestive issues, pain, or difficulties with your skin? You recently erred from your healthier routines? maybe it's time to cleanse.

Detoxifying may help cover you from complaint, restore your energy to maintain optimal health, help you lose weight, and cover you from complaint by clearing your body of   poisons and also furnishing it with healthy nutrients.

Detoxification is simply the process of sanctifying the blood. In the liver, where   poisons are reused for excretion, it primarily accomplishes this by barring contaminations from the rotation. The   feathers, intestine, lungs, lymph, and epidermis are other organs that the body uses to get   relieve of   poisons. Every cell in the body suffers when this system is damaged because contaminations aren't   rightly filtered.

A detox program may support the body's   essential cleaning procedure by:

1) giving the organs a break;

2) encouraging the liver to remove poisons from the body;

3) perfecting elimination through the skin,   feathers, and

intestine;

4) perfecting blood rotation; and

5) refueling the body with healthy nutrients.

A minimum of   formerly per time, you ought to cleanse. Generally speaking, a light detoxifying authority is safe; in fact, exploration show that a detox is good for your health.However, a   sprat, or a person who has cancer or tuberculosis, If you're a nursing mother.However, speak with your croaker, If you are doubtful about whether sanctification is right for you. Reduce your poison burden at first. Remove all poisons from your system, including booze, coffee, cigarettes, sugar, and concentrated fats, which can obstruct the mending process. Reduce the use of   particular care particulars and ménage cleansers with chemicals and switch to organic druthers

.

Stress is another obstacle to good health because it causes your body to produce stress hormones. While these hormones may give you the "adrenaline rush" you need to win a race or finish a task on time, excessive quantities of them also create toxins, slow down the liver's detoxification enzymes, and may even make you gain weight.

Consequently, it makes sense to detoxify your body and your stressful life circumstances at the same time. By resetting your physical and mental reactions to the unavoidable tension life will bring, yoga and meditation are easy and effective ways to relieve tension.

Various detoxification programs are available, based on your unique needs. Many programs follow a 7-day schedule because it calls for a 2-day liquid fast followed by a carefully thought-out 5-day diet to give the digestive system time to recover. To improve circulation, experts suggest using vitamins, herbs, physical activity, and techniques like hydrotherapy and dry skin brushing.

A 3 – 7 day liquid fast is also a successful method of

detoxification. A different option is purifying supplement packets, which typically include fiber, vitamins, herbs, and minerals. There are many trustworthy goods with simple to understand instructions available on the market. One day a week of drinking nothing but water is a long-standing custom in many societies.

Following a detox program, you can cleanse your body every day through food, supplements, and lifestyle changes, which helps you maintain a healthy weight.

1. Consume a lot of fiber, such as that found in brown rice and freshly grown organic fruits and vegetables. Excellent detoxifying meals include beets, radishes, artichokes, cabbage, broccoli, spirulina, chlorella, and seaweed.

2. Drink green tea and take herbs like milk thistle, burdock, and dandelion root to cleanse and protect the liver.

3. Consume vitamin C, which aids in the body's production of glutathione, a liver compound that eliminates toxins.

4. Drink two quarts or more of water every day.

5. Take a few deep breaths to allow your body to absorb oxygen more completely.

6. Reduce tension by focusing on uplifting feelings.

7. Use hydrotherapy by taking a brief, extremely warm shower and allowing the water to flow down your back. Follow up with 30 seconds of cool water. Then, after three repetitions, lie down for 30 minutes.

8. Sweat in a sauna to help your body eliminate wastes through perspiration.

9. To expel toxins through your pores, dry brush your skin, use detoxifying patches, or take detox foot baths. Natural goods stores sell specialized brushes.

Be sure to speak with your doctor before beginning any new regimen.

CHAPTER 3

Synopsis

Along with helping people lose weight, harmonious exertion has a number of other proven, positive health benefits, particularly for their hearts. The heart becomes a bigger, more important muscle after vigorous exercise, strengthening it as a pump.

Indeed moderate exercise can ameliorate rotation, lower blood pressure, and lower blood fat situations while adding HDL (the "good" cholesterol). Reduced threat for heart complaint, heart attacks, rotundity, and stroke is the result of all these goods.

Get Moving Advantages

Along with helping you keep a healthy weight, being active may also offer benefits like strengthened muscles, bettered inflexibility, and stronger bones, which may help shield off the bone- thinning physical condition known as osteoporosis.

Regular exercise also guarantees positive goods on internal health, similar as lowering anxiety and melancholy. You might get further rest and have further vitality as a result. Exercise would be the most popular catholicon at the neighborhood drugstore if it could be packaged.

Everyone should exercise. nearly everyone can profit from exercise in terms of their good. But checks every many times confirm the well- known verity that utmost people are not physically fit enough. sorely, we've to pay for it. About 250,000 losses per time in the United States, or 13 of all deaths, are attributed by the American Heart Association to inactivity. Chancing the reasons for inactivity isn't delicate.

It's rare for utmost of us to engage in physical exertion at work because utmost of our jobs bear us to lay down utmost of the time. In order to avoid homemade labor, we also heavily depend on ultramodern, labor- saving technologies like buses , appliances, and power tools.

Still, there's another reason why numerous people, especially the   fat, avoid physical exercise. Look at the toned, athletic numbers displayed working out on TV or magazine covers. They convey the idea that working out is sweaty, delicate labor stylish left to the youthful, physically fit, and athletic. ultramodern study,   still, shows that this perception is untrue and that benefits can still be   attained from low- intensity exertion,   similar as gardening.

You'll lose weight if you expend further calories than you consume. You'll lose one pound for every fresh,500 calories that you consume. Exercise hard, and you will expend calories snappily. also, you can burn the same quantum of calories with simpler exercise. Just do it more frequently and/ or for an extended period of time. However, you may find it discouraging when you first learn about it, If you're strange with how numerous calories are consumed during exercise. For illustration, if you weigh 150 pounds and walk hastily for 20 twinkles on a afar, you will burn about 100 calories, which is significantly lower than the 500 calories demanded to lose a pound. Still, you will have a 3,500- calorie deficiency by the end of the week.

If you burn an redundant 300 calories per day through physical exertion and cut 200 calories from your diet. This exact kind of gradational success is what specialists recommend for long-term weight control. also, physical exercise helps the body lose weight. It develops strength and eliminates fat. Muscle weighs further than fat does for a particular mass. thus, indeed though your bath scale may not show significant changes, your apparel will be looser and your body form will be slender.

As exercise builds muscle, it may also help neutralize a problem brought on by eating. Your body's metabolism may decelerate down and consume calories more sluggishly when you cut back on calories. This makes farther weight reduction more delicate. still, some study suggests that regular exercise can help to overcome this pause and   grease weight loss.

Your body may break down muscle as a result of weight loss from reducing calories without exercise, which eventually slows down your metabolism and makes losing weight more delicate. When people stop eating healthy, the problem of calorie restriction without exercise becomes more serious. They constantly recover all of their lost weight and   also some because they've lost muscle.

A superior strategy is to increase your physical exertion, which helps you   make muscle, while reducing your calorie input from food. Exercise can help you manage your stress situations and regulate your appetite, which can help you repel the temptation to binge.

Combing leaves or playing a videotape game both demand energy, but how important depends on 3 effects your muscle mass, your body weight, and the exertion itself. The further body   corridor you move that are heavier and have further muscular mass, the further calories you burn. Exercise frequency, intensity, and length all factor into weight loss. .

CHAPTER 4

__Figure Out When You Start To Burn Fat__

Synopsis

The highly contentious "fat burning zone" refers to the target pulse rate range that is meant to aid weight loss. About 60% of the calories you expend during low-intensity, prolonged exercise come from fat, not carbohydrates.

Only about 35% of the calories burned during intense activity come from fat. Exercise physiologists claim that low-intensity exercise does help people lose weight. Simply do it for a longer amount of time.

Where Is The Zone

Alternating between low-intensity and high-intensity physical activity is best for the body's health because it promotes healing, optimal wellness, and rapid weight reduction that most people would find acceptable.

Sprinters, to put it simply, have that appearance of muscle on muscle, whereas the average treadmill walker has thin arms and a gut? It's simple. When you sprint, you put your muscles through such intense strain that they grow larger and stronger as a result. Therefore, combining the fat-burning zone with workouts of greater intensity will produce the outcomes that the majority of people are looking for.

For the maximum goal pulse rate for the fat burning zone, start with 180 minus your age (a) (z). $180 - a = z$ is the solution.

Take your heart rate (p) for 15 seconds while exercising, then increase it by four to get your pulse rate (h) for one minute. This is the heart rate you experience while working out or exercising. In this case, (p) times 15 sec = h.

Stay in the fat-burning region. Your heart rate must remain within or at the z (upper pulse rate limit during conditioning for the fat burning zone) determined in Step 1. Numerous exercise devices have calculations that, based on your age, will give you a range (the zone—an upper and lower limit).

Additional calculations:

Establish your MHR (Age Predicted Maximum Heart Rate). MHR Equals 220 less your current age.

Calculate your RHR (Resting Heart Rate). Take your heart rate (p) for 15 seconds when you first wake up or when you are completely relaxed. Then, multiply that number by 4 to get your resting pulse rate for one minute.

Input your MHR and RHR using 85% of the calculation. 65% to 85% can be used to create a fat-burning zone.

Fill in (percent of max) with 85% for the top of your fat-burning zone and (percent of max) with 65% or 75% for the bottom of your fat-burning zone. You now know the zone or range of your activity that will burn the most fat.

To get the most benefit from exercise, including bettering cardiovascular health, burning fat, improving flexibility, and toning and conditioning the body, mix up your workouts by incorporating extended, low-intensity physical activity as well as short, high-intensity workouts.

Before starting a new diet or weight loss plan, always seek the counsel and advice of a licensed doctor. This includes figuring out the ideal fat-burning zone or target heart rate.

CHAPTER 5

Easy Ways To Eat Healthy

Synopsis

It doesn't have to be a drastic change to eat healthier and lose weight. Here are some easy steps to adopt healthy eating habits. You don't have to totally give up the foods that you enjoy eating. These are merely methods for reducing extra calories.

Simple Healthy Eating

***   Stop consuming SodaPop pop or energy   potables with high calorie counts.**

By drinking soda pop pop, you incontinently gain weight that you wouldn't have if you had not indulged in the effervescent drinks from the dealing machine. Water should be used in place of those   potables. Adding bomb or cucumber slices to your drink will help you get used to the taste if you are put off by water's mellow flavor. However, plain water won't be as amping , If flavor is introduced.

*** Consume water when you feel empty.**

It's possible that you are confusing appetite with thirst. You might find that drinking water makes you feel full and prevents you from looking for junk food.

*** Figure a ornamental fruit arrangement for your home that's filled with real fruit.**

Buy a gorgeous coliseum to display your fresh yield in. For accessible access, put it in the kitchen. You'll be drawn to it, which will beget you to consume a lot of fruit. Encourage your entire family to join you in getting gooey by keeping it full at all times.

* <u>Shift to 100 percent whole wheat food</u>.

To make whole wheat chuck , pasta, crackers, and cereal more charming to your taste receptors, it's simple to do.

* <u>Do not adulation your food.</u>

Without   fresh adulation, some foods, like vegetables, may taste excellent. Enjoy its wholesome tastiness in the purest form. Try the spread adulation if you need to gradationally transition to this change. Per drop, there are   generally only a many calories.

* <u>Stand back from frozen foods which may be high in sodium.</u>

Check the sodium   position on the marker whenever you buy

any kind of reused food. You can ameliorate your health and reduce your circumference if you just take the time to prepare your own   refections rather than buying frozen bones

* <u>Do not add fresh swab to your food.</u>

utmost foods   formerly contain a lot of   swab, which can beget clogged   highways. Add a variety of spices to your mess to give it   redundant flavor. Without any   redundant fat, you   will   get   a   full   flavor   from   this.

Wrapping Up

Maintaining your body in peak physical condition is only one aspect of staying healthy. It's also extremely important to maintain good brain wellness. There are many things you can do on a daily basis to maintain a beautiful and healthy intellect and body.

Studying comes first. Yes, I am aware that most people dislike studying in their spare time, but it is essential to maintaining mental acuity. Studying strengthens your brain by regularly supplying it with information and cerebral exercise. Spend some time reading every day. It doesn't matter what you're studying; it could be a 500-page book or a magazine.

Find a stress-relieving activity is the second thing to do. It could be watching a video, going swimming, or just spending some time with your kids. When it's feasible, set aside some time to engage in a particular daily action that relieves stress.

The effects of stress on the body are severe and may even

contribute to its demise.

This is really, really bad for your health if you smoke and drink. It's crucial to take care of your health, and these bad habits will only harm it.

It will probably be one of the toughest things to break these habits, but it will be worthwhile in the end.

Finally, remember to always smile and have a positive perspective on life. Try to find the positive side of every circumstance, even if it seems impossible.

If you have to do something during the day that you find horrible, just tell yourself it's something to look forward to. Daily smiles not only improve your mood but also inspire others.

These are just a few suggestions for keeping your body and

intellect healthy. Finding what works best for you only requires a little effort.

Remember that getting fit doesn't have to be a drawn-out, challenging mental procedure. Personal goals are not difficult to accomplish, even on a small scale, if given the proper information and assistance. Living a healthy lifestyle can be very gratifying and can help you keep a healthy weight without having to diet all the time.